Wheat Belly Diet

Grain Brain Eating

By Cathy Wilson

Copyright © 2014

Income Disclaimer

This book contains business strategies, marketing methods and other business advice that, regardless of my own results and experience, may not produce the same results (or any results) for you. I make absolutely no guarantee, expressed or implied, that by following the advice below you will make any money or improve current profits, as there are several factors and variables that come into play regarding any given business.

Primarily, results will depend on the nature of the product or business model, the conditions of the marketplace, the experience of the individual, and situations and elements that are beyond your control.

As with any business endeavor, you assume all risk related to investment and money based on your own discretion and at your own potential expense.

Liability Disclaimer

By reading this book, you assume all risks associated with using the advice given below, with a full understanding that you, solely, are responsible for anything that may occur as a result of putting this information into action in any way, and regardless of your interpretation of the advice.

You further agree that our company cannot be held responsible in any way for the success or failure of your business as a result of the information presented in this book. It is your responsibility to conduct your own due diligence regarding the safe and successful operation of your business if you intend to apply any of our information in any way to your business operations.

Terms of Use

Wheat Belly Diet
Grain Brain Eating

By Cathy Wilson

Table of Contents

Introduction

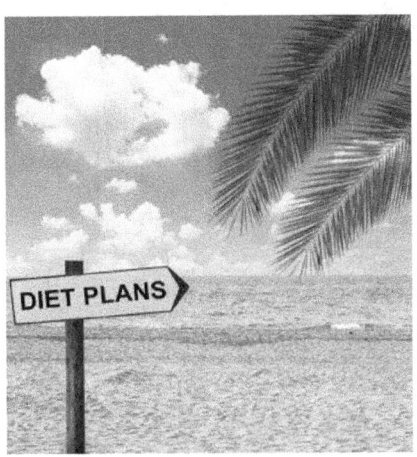

Losing weight isn't easy. By **COMMITTING** to make the eating changes necessary to blast fat, you're taking your first step toward reaching your health and wellness goals.

FACT - Dr. William Davis, cardiologist, published the infamous Wheat Belly diet book in 2001. And from that point gluten-free, or wheat-free eating, has made headlines.

This introductory book is all about providing you with practical information to help you lose fat and get healthy. Featuring the Wheat Belly Diet.

FACT - Not every diet plan will work for everyone!

I'm a firm believer there is no ONE diet plan that works for anyone forever. Staying healthy is all about change. This means as new scientific information comes in, what you eat, when, and how much, gets adjusted.

There are fantabulous facts about wheat-free eating that can help you lose weight. Particularly if you're eating nutrition-less, high fat, high sugar bad "grain" carbohydrates. There's a gynormous difference between choosing to eat processed and refined wheat grain products, and all-natural unprocessed organic wheat products.

This book uses scientific opinion to make factual clarifications that will help you determine if all, of any part of the Wheat Belly Diet concept is the right move for you!

Chapter One - Wheat Belly Basics

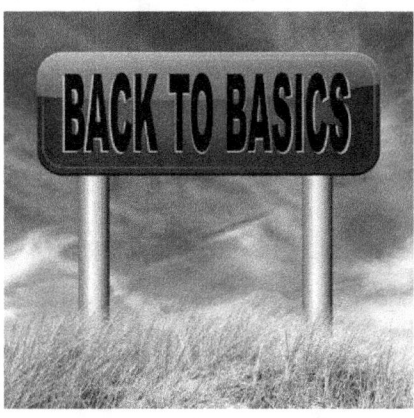

This Wheat Belly diet concept was created by MD William Davis, in hopes of preventing weight gain and serious disease.

GOAL - To achieve *PERMANENT* weight loss and prevent or reduce the effects of a wide range of health issues, from immune system disorders, to digestive problems, and arthritis.

THE BELIEF - People aren't fat because they don't exercise and eat high-fat, junky, processed fast foods, it's because they're eating wheat! Found in cakes, muffins, pasta, bread, and pastries.

CIP - Cathy's Important Point - Although I agree and support most of what the wheat belly diet is aiming to accomplish, I don't agree completely with *the belief* behind this diet.

TRUTH - High-fat wheat foods will trigger weight gain

FALSE - Lack of exercise and crap food choices don't contribute to getting fat!

Health Harvard reports 60% of U.S adults are overweight, and one-third of American adults are obese. And the US government recommends at least an hour of vigorous exercise a day. I'm sure they aren't saying that just for the fun of it!

National Heart, Lung, and Blood Institute reports an inactive lifestyle raises the risk for heart disease, high blood pressure, colon cancer, diabetes, and various other health issues. Lack of exercise also triggers weight gain.

According to *NHS Choices*, obesity is generally caused by moving too little and eating too much.

*Increasing your energy output through routine intense exercise, will only increase your calories used, speeding up the process in which you lose weight, when combined with healthy eating.

Chapter Two - Cons of Wheat

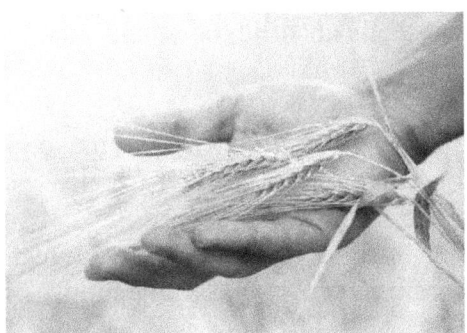

According to the Wheat Belly Diet Concept, there are quite a few health dangers interconnected with wheat containing foods.

*STORING FAT and INSULIN RESPONSE

Wheat triggers insulin response which encourages fat storage. Research studies show that fat gain tends to be in the belly area. What's interesting, is that wheat catalyzes endorphin release. This gives you that "feel good feeling," and boots your appetite so you want to eat more.

Process of Carbohydrate and Blood Sugar Breakdown

According to *Harvard School of Public Health*, when you eat foods containing carbohydrates, like wheat, your digestive systems breaks down useable ones into sugars, and these sugars enter your blood for energy use.

Fact - When your blood sugars rise, the pancreas manufactures insulin. This hormone tells your cells to absorb these sugars for energy, and/or put them into storage.

Fact - When your cells absorb blood sugar, the blood sugar levels drop.

Fact - This drop signals your pancreas to make glucugaon. And this hormone then tells your liver to release sugar stores.

Fact - It's the responsibility of glucagon and insulin to ensure your body and brain have a good steady supply of glucose in the blood.

Wheat is a carbohydrate that's unique in structure. Technically it's made of seventy-five percent amylopectin and twenty-five percent amylose. Which is stressful for blood sugar regulation.

Everything you eat influences blood glucose levels. And because of wheat's specific composition, the response to your blood sugar levels is more severe.

*GLUTEN

Peter H.R. Green, MD, Columbia University Celiac Disease Center director, says people with celiac disease must eat gluten-free. But for most others, the concern with a gluten-free diet, is the lack of essential vitamins, minerals, and fiber.

Just reminds you there are two sides to every story. Figure out what works for you and move forward positively.

Wheat has this gluten protein that causes celiac disease, which is labelled the most common *missed* wheat allergy.

Gluten is also linked to...

14

*Gastrointestinal disease

*Arthritis

*IBS

*Yeast infections

*Neurological issues

More Reasons to Ponder Avoiding Wheat

*_Paleo Leap_ reports up to eighty percent of the population gets an inflamed gut from gluten. Up to thirty percent in unable to process gluten proteins.

*Gliadin is a gluten protein that causes issues. It's similar to other proteins in your organs, and can trigger antibodies against gliadin to go after these organs. This causes autoimmune issues, including diabetes and hypothyroidism.

*Because of the swelling caused by gluten, gut cells may die early, creating oxidization. This evolves into a leaky gut, enabling bacterias and toxins into your blood stream, which of course is dangerous. Not to mention the inability to absorb all the essential vitamins and minerals your body needs.

*Some studies show that gluten antibodies can attack the heart.

*Research shows gluten is directly linked with various types of cancer.

*The opioid peptides in wheat trigger wheat addiction. Meaning when people remove wheat from their diet they may experience unpleasant side effects.

*Studies show when Schizophrenia patients take wheat out of their diet, their symptoms improve tremendously. Some experts go so far as to say that wheat triggers this disease.

My Thoughts...

Recent research studies seem to support the negatives of including wheat in your diet. I use the term loosely because there are types of wheat that are considerably more taxing on your health than others. We'll cover that a few chapters down the road.

What you've gotta do is work with your healthcare provider, and figure out if the negative effects of wheat on your health, are worth removing them, and to what degree.

Next up's the flip side of the coin...

Chapter Three - Wheat Benefits

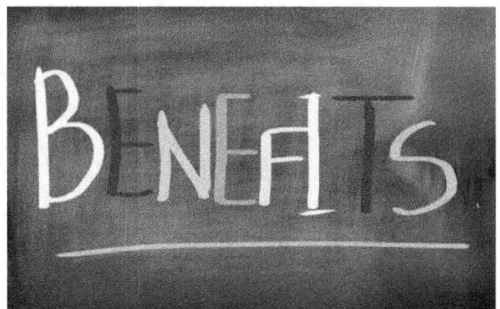

The first red flag that should make you skeptical about a particular diet, is when a component of it is only discussed negatively. Just about everything in life has pluses and minuses, even deadly trans fat!

One positive of *trans fat* is there are minute amounts that occur naturally in animal products. Although unless you're visibly eating the fat off the edge of a T-bone steak, it won't hurt you. In fact, according to far experts Sally Fallon and Mary Enig, the natural trans fat vaccenic acid, VD, appears to help battle cancer. Keep in mind, there are no *safe* levels of natural trans fat.

Fact - Wheat is the most common cereal in the world.

Wheat originated in southwestern Asia, and is readily used to make bagels, cakes, pasta, bread, crackers, and muffins.

Fact - *Organic Facts* reports wheat is one of the most wholesome foods. Rich in fiber and vital nutrients.

Wheat Nutrition

Wheat has oodles of nutrition, including: sulfur, chlorine, magnesium, mineral salts, calcium, arsenic, manganese, silicon, vitamin E and D, copper, iodide, and zinc.

Wheat's recommended to treat sterility. And a whole whack of health issues improve with wheat nutrients, like anemia, pregnancy problems, gallstones, and mineral deficiencies.

Wheat Benefits

*Controls Obesity - Particularly in Women - The *American Journal of Clinical Nutrition* reports, whole wheat foods consumed over long periods of time by women, showed a larger amount of weight loss than the other subjects. It's also believed wheat has the natural ability to control weight in everyone.

*Prevents Diabetes - Magnesium found in wheat, acts as a co-factor for more than 300 enzymes. What's critical, is these enzymes are involved in glucose secretion and the body's use of insulin.

FDA FACT - Whole grain food by a minimum 51% weight, are low in cholesterol and saturated fat. This means a lower risk of various cancers and heart issues.

Add to that, regular whole grain consumption levels blood sugar. For diabetics, replacing rice with wheat regulates blood glucose levels.

*Boosts Metabolism - Wheat is very effective on people with metabolic issues.

Metabolic Disorders:

-Visceral obesity - pear shape

-Low levels HDL cholesterol (protective)

-High blood fat

-Elevated blood pressure

Wheat helps protect against metabolic disorders.

Experts agree, the fiber in wheat products helps the digestive process and improves metabolism.

*Deters Gallstones - According to the *American Journal of Gastroenterology*, wheat products help women avoid gall-stones.

Why?

Wheat's rich in insoluble fiber. This ensures quick movement internally, with less bile acid produced. Eating lots of wheat also boosts insulin sensitivity, lowering fat in your blood.

Other sources of insoluble fiber are...

-Apples
-Pears
-Cucumbers
-Berries
-Squash
-Tomatoes
-Beans

*Helps Prevent Disease - According to *Organic Facts*, three cups of wheat each day is plenty to ensure waste is pushed through your system, so you can live a long life free of disease.

*Lowers Risk for Chronic Inflammation - Betanine is found in spinach, beets, and wheat. It help to prevent internal swelling.

Keeping inflammation down in your body decreases the risk of developing diabetes, cardiovascular disease, bone degeneration, Alzheimer's, and mental breakdown.

Reduces Risk of Breast Cancer - According to *Cancer Research UK*, there's evidence that diets with more than 25 grams of fiber reduces the risk of breast cancer in pre-menopausal women. Whole grain wheat, fruits and veggies, are all high in fiber.

Postmenopausal Women have Improved Cardio Function - A diet high in wheat slows down the manifestation of atherosclerosis, or hardening of the arteries that often leads to stroke or heart attack.

VIP NOTE - There can be too much of a good thing! Wheat has oxalates. These occur naturally in humans, plants, and animals. Problem is, too much of these oxalates will trigger crystallization. This can cause minor health issues like kidney stones, gout, and gallstones.

MODERATION IS KEY IN EVERYTHING!

My Thoughts...

That's a heck of a lot of votes for the wheat side of the equation. Just keep your mind open to everything, and figure out what works best for you. Obviously if you've a wheat allergy,

20

minor or major, gluten-free is your route. And the Wheat Belly Diet is your route to losing fat and building your health strong.

The benefits of including healthy wheat in your diet is a gy-normous positive, so don't be afraid to include them. You'll more likely find your balance taking the basic concepts of the Wheat Belly Diet, and modifying them to fit with YOUR personal preferences and tolerances.

Lots to consider, so let's keep going.

Chapter Four - Modern Day Wheat

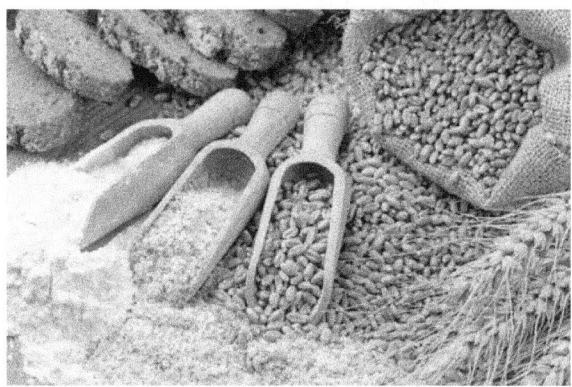

The issue with wheat is QUALITY. There's a gynormous difference between the healthy whole grains people ate directly from Mother Nature centuries ago, and a lot of the refined processed crap we eat today.

In fact, our fast-paced world caters to clever marketing campaigns and sensationalizing fast foods, to make people *THINK* they're eating whole grains, when really it's just a bunch of nutrition-less, vitamin and mineral stripped naked crap!

TRUTH - What once was an ancient food staple, has transformed into toxic crap junk!

FACT - Grain has been a healthy staple food since the beginning of time. It's readily available, stores for long periods of time, and releases fantabulous amounts of healthy nutrition when prepared in hot cereals, breads, and clean eating baked goods.

According to *Grainstorm*, for over 10,000 years humans have relied on this healthy wheat product for survival.

WHAT HAPPENED??

What Changed?

*The way we eat it
*The way we grow it
*The way we process it
*The wheat itself

PROCESSING

Manufacturers started processing wheat and the rest is history! White flour was discovered in the late 1800s, by beating the crap out of the wheat. This created a market for white flour, which could be sold cheap.

So freshness is lost with processing. And manufacturers continued to break down the base product and look for ways to get more for less, make it store longer, and essentially get more bang for their buck!

As the processing component progressed, the vital minerals and nutrients of the once healthy wheat product went straight out the window.

White bread, pasta, and rice is sweet. People are naturally drawn to it. Over time you've been taught to accept and even crave processed wheat products, which are the triggers for serious health issues. If we were talking about REAL wheat, unprocessed from centuries ago, the story would be totally different.

DEMAND FOR MORE

Humans always want more for less. With wheat there were radical genetic modifications made, producing high-input farming. This meant various fertilizers and pesticides were used to increase the wheat produced.

That's all find and dandy, but what about the QUALITY?

Scientists took from nature, rearranged all the internal components, and pumped out a totally fake and unhealthy produced, and called it WHEAT.

Fake soil, fake seeds, fake environment, fake growing condition...YIKES!

IS YOUR HEALTH WORTH SAVING A FEW BUCKS FOR MORE?

There's a difference between Gluten Intolerance, and Wheat Sensitivity

GLUTEN INTOLERANCE - Means you can't have any gluten at all without serious consequences. An itty-bitty percentage of the population falls here.

WHEAT SENSITIVITY - Means something in modern day wheat triggers mild issues for you. Something that likely wouldn't be an issue if you were consuming REAL wheat in centuries past.

Now you've got to fiddle-faddle around to try and figure out what modified versions of wheat products suit you, and which ones don't!

BEWARE - CRAP GLUTEN-FREE FOODS!

Careful where you step...

There are oodles of gluten-free foods that are complete junk.
So make sure you read the label carefully.

*Cornstarch
*Tapioca starch
*Rice starch
*Potato starch
*Guar gum

Each of these are often substituted for white flour, and many
are worse than white sugar for spiking your blood glucose levels!

SOLUTION: Try organic and stone ground wheat, minus all
the crap processing and additives.

Healthy Flour Facts

You'd think *whole wheat* is healthy. But in most cases it's not.
Technically white flour with a little bit of bran thrown in to
disguise it, can be called *whole wheat.*

*CIP - Cathy's Important Point - *Search for STONE
GROUND WHOLE WHEAT FLOUR. Where the entire ker-
nel is crushed and kept together, not separated and
substituted.*

This natural grain doesn't store long, and breaks down quickly.
Which obviously doesn't make it an ideal ingredient for any
sort of foods mass produced on the grocery shelf.

**COWS ARE SMARTER THAN WE ARE! AND TRUST
ME, THEY'RE PRETTY FREAKIN DUMB! :)**

I grew up on a farm. My cows wouldn't eat their grain if it
wasn't fresh. I knew this because you could smell the acid scent

it gave off it too many nutrients were lost, and it was just plain old stale. The cows would look at me with their big brown eyes, wondering why the hell I'm trying to feed them crap grain!

They preferred the fresh ground chop and so should we!

NASTY INGREDIENTS IN PROCESSED BREADS

According to *Natural Savvy*, here are a few of the chemical additives you'll find in processed bread products.

Calcium peroxide - banned in China
Chlorine and chlorine dioxide gas - banned in EU
Benzoyl peroxide - banned in both EU and China
Calcium bromate and Azodicarbonamide - banned in EU and Canada
Nitrogen dioxide and potassium bromate - banned in China, Canada, Nigeria+++

Holy Crap! If that's not enough to make you think twice about eating unnatural processed wheat, I don't know what is!

Health Dangers of Processed Wheat and Grains

*Spike Blood Sugars - Processed wheat offered fast energy that spikes your blood sugars. This large dose of sugar creates free radicals that damages proteins, making your tissues age faster.

*Too many carbs - History dictates ancient man got 98 percent of their carbohydrates from fruits and veggies. Need I say more?

*Triggers Insulin Spike - When excess refined sugars enter your blood, the body naturally increases insulin levels. Your pancreas gets overworked producing the insulin, which enables your cells to use the glucose for energy. When too much insulin is produced, your cells start to reject it. Which of course creates a whole new whack of health issues for you.

Some of which are...

-Diabetes
-Obesity
-Cardiovascular disease
-Blood pressure issues
-Alzheimer's
-Dementia
-Cancers

*Crap Nutrients and Little Fiber - Modern day wheat grains have been processed and refined to the max. They're left with very little nutrients and next to no fiber.

*Watch for Phytates - Whole grains contain phytates, which can interfere with the absorption of magnesium and zinc. Both of which are critical for a restful sleep. Check out *Livestrong* for more.

*Watch for the Lectins - Processed whole grains have lectins that enable more junk to get into your body via the blood. Lectins are confusing to your blood because some of the crap getting into your blood looks like proteins, and starts attacking the crap and proteins. This causes everything from simple skin issues to MS.

Lectins in their natural form are meant to pass into your system undisturbed and unaltered, not to alert your immune system. When grain products are refined and the lectins are screwed around with, this red flags your immune system response and creates all the trouble!

LECTINS natural and in moderation are good.

28

LECTINS in excess and modified, like in processed wheat, are NAUGHTY!

My Thoughts...

You can see there's a gynormous difference between healthy REAL wheat, and the processed refined crap we eat today. Fooling around with the internal composition of any food is dangerous. Adding chemicals, preservatives, and other toxic substances is plain old KILLER.

Science says there's really nothing healthy about modern day wheat. Time for you to take this fact and do something with it. You deserve to live clean and healthy!

Chapter Five - Health Benefits of Wheat Belly Diet

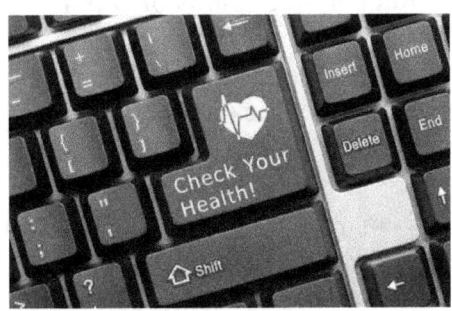

WebMD states the Wheat Belly Diet claims to help you drop fat, feel more positive, and have more energy! Sounds fantabulous to me!

Academy of Nutrition and Dietetics, the world's largest organization of food and nutrition professionals, has a few interesting things to say about *Wheat Belly*.

This eating plan is simple and complex simultaneously. It's got only ONE hard-fast rule. Which is to eliminate ALL forms of wheat. The complex part is that a large portion of what we eat contains wheat and wheat products, both hidden and obvious, natural and processed.

Keep in mind, many of the substitutions or alternatives to wheat in products, is just as unhealthy as or worse than the wheat. Rice and potato flour are often used in gluten-free products in place of wheat, and they're both nasty for your health, particularly in spiking your blood glucose levels.

Tough Nut to Swallow - This diet calls for just 50-100 grams of carbs per day.

*1 cup of grapes has 39 grams of carbs
*1/2 cup of chickpeas has 25grams of carbs
*1 cup of squash has 30 grams of carbs
*1 cup of orange juice has 25 grams of carbs
*1/2 cup of pasta has 30 grams of carbs
*4 Saltine crackers has 15 grams of carbs
*2 small chocolate chip cookies has 15 grams of carbs
*1 cup cereal has 30 grams of carbs

You can see how easy it is to overdose easily with your carbs in just one sitting!!

Dr. Davis mentions you shouldn't need any supplements for vitamins and minerals lost, with the appropriate substitutions. Unfortunately there aren't a lot of healthy substitutions to replace the vitamins and minerals lost.

The experts at the *Academy of Nutrition and Dietetics* suggests going through this plan with a registered dietician because otherwise you may be seriously deficient in B vitamins, vitamin D, and calcium, to name a few.

 VIP - Dr. Davis also recommends not substituting foods like rice and potato flour, because they increase the metabolic response. But by eliminating these starches from your diet you would theoretically lose weight anyway. Which raises the question, are you losing weight because you're eliminating wheat, or carbohydrates?

Bottom line is, this group of specialists have the same thoughts as I do. The average American is gonna have a hell of a time sticking to this rather restrictive diet, and find healthy substitutions for wheat foods.

According to *Chewfo*, promoting the Wheat Belly Diet, there's a huge list of health benefits with this eating plan, including reducing the risk of...

*Autism
*Bloating
*Brain fog
*Breast cancer
*Acne
*Skin issues
*ADHD
*Asthma and other breathing issues
*Bowel issues
*Cardiovascular disease
*Dementia
*Alzheimer's
*Diabetes
*Cancers
*Penis issues
*Kidney disease
*Flatulence
*Obesity
*Food addiction
*Bone disease
*PH imbalance
*Various types of arthritis
*Ulcers
*Wrinkles
*Psoriasis

CIP - Cathy's Important Point - Do not start any sort of new eating strategy without first discussing it with your healthcare provider. Better safe than sorry!

My Thoughts...

People that are successful in long-term weight loss, set up reasonable expectations with their eating plan, exercise routine, a lifestyle parameters. Your good health is multifactorial. A balance of healthy changes that YOU can stick with.

Yes, you can lose fat on the Wheat Belly Diet. But you can also do it ten zillion other ways that may be easier for you.

Chapter Six - Wheat Foods You Can and Can't Eat and Shortcomings

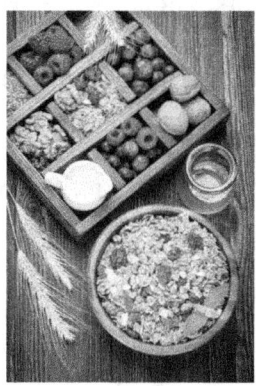

With the Wheat Belly Diet you've gotta eliminate all wheat. This includes bread, pasta, pretzels, donuts, muffins, cakes, pretzels, etc. Toss into all that, foods made with spelt, barley, some oats, rye and wheat, according to *WebMd*.

*This is a low-carb eating strategy where you avoid bad fat and cured meats.

BEWARE - This doesn't mean you can substitute *GLUTEN-FREE* for everything. Many of these foods, as we've mentioned before, have cornstarch, rice starch, tapioca starch, and potato starch that trigger the same dangerous blood glucose spike.

Also make a note of removing sugary foods, excess salt, sucrose, corn syrup, pop, potatoes, and fruit juice. Fried foods and trans fat foods shouldn't even be in your vocabulary.

EAT AND ENJOY:

Veggies - a variety of organic if possible

*Prime choice - squash, carrots, broccoli, peppers, avocado, beans, kale, eggplant, leeks, onions, mushrooms, sprouts, cucumber, dandelions, radishes, tomatoes, spinach, peas, scallions, water chestnuts, zucchini, celery

Dairy products - choose organic if possible

*Full-fat cheese - edam, feta, goat cheese, mozzarella, Monterey Jack, cheddar, Comte, swiss, ricotta, parmesan, provolone

Fish and shellfish

*Fish - cod, snapper, perch, bass, salmon, tuna, red snapper
*Shellfish plus - scallops, shrimp, lobster, clams, crab, oysters

Meat and poultry

*Try to buy organic and grass-fed
*Unprocessed
*Meats - buffalo, beef, wild game, veal, beef, pork, lamb
*Poultry - turkey, pheasant, chicken, duck, quail
*Canadian bacon
*Uncured sausage and turkey bacon
*No high-fat cooking, like frying in grease!

Eggs

*Any way you like them!

Fats

*Use healthy unsaturated oils
*Avocado oil, extra virgin olive oil, flaxseed oil, almond oil, peanut oil, sesame oil

*Organic butter
*Coconut oil
*Cook at low temperatures and don't fry!

Raw nuts/seeds

*Almonds, cashews, peanuts, macadamias, coconut, Brazil nuts, hazelnuts, walnuts, pecans
*Keep in mind nuts are high in fat and calories - 1/4 cup is a serving!
*Flaxseed, sunflower seeds, sesame seeds, poppy seeds,
*Almond butter, nut butter, peanut butter, sunflower butter

Flour substitutes

*Needs to be gluten-free and wheat-free
*Read ingredients to make sure there's no carb crap substitutions, like potato starch, cornstarch, and rice starch
*Almond flour, almond meal, coconut flour, ground flaxseed, pumpkin seed flour, sunflower seed meal, walnut meal
*Store in sealed container in freezer or fridge to help prevent oxidization
*Keep in fridge no more than a few days
*Keep in freezer no more than a few weeks

Herbs and spices

*Anise, chives, basil, bay leaf, sage, rosemary, cilantro, thyme, tarragon, parsley, mint, dill
*Chili powder, allspice, cinnamon, coriander, celery seed, paprika, wasabi, salt, saffron, cumin, fennel

*Pretty much any herb or spice works

Sweeteners

*Splenda, stevia, xylitol, erythritol

Drinks

*Water
*Tea
*Coconut milk, almond milk
*Coconut water
*Coffee

Condiments

*Avoid sugary choices
*Chili sauces, salsa, mustards, vinegars, Worcestershire sauce, tamara, salsa, fish sauce, mayo

Extras

*Lemons, limes
*Beef or chicken broth, coconut milk canned, tomato paste, tomato juice
*Pickled - olives, veggies, sauerkraut
*Baking - baking powder, baking soda, arrowroot, cocoa powder

EAT IN MODERATION:

Non-Cheese dairy

*Organic
*Half and half, cream, milk, sour cream
*Fresh Cheese - cream cheese, cottage cheese
*Yogurts - unsweetened and flavored
*Buttermilk
*Kefir
*Full-fat dairy, unprocessed if possible

Fruit

*Organic
*All berries
*Limited apples, pears, apricots, oranges
*Steer clear of sugary fruits like pineapple, bananas, mango, papaya
*Fruit juices
*Unsweetened applesauce - watch sugar
*Dried fruit

Non-gluten grains, non-wheat

*1/2 cup less serving
*Chia seeds, millet, oats, teff, wild rice, amaranth
*Rice, corn - too many nutrients stripped with genetic alterations

Legumes

*Limit to 1/2 cup serving
*All beans
*Chickpeas
*Lentils
*Carob
*Peanuts - not raw, boiled or roasted
*Soybeans

Starchy Veggies

*Whole corn
*All potatoes

Drinks

*Wheat-free alcohol - limit 1-2 glasses/week wine or cocktail

Other

*Semi-sweet chocolate

Foods to Avoid:

*Gluten grains
*Wheat-based baked goods
*Gluten foods like baquettes, burritos, couscous, croutons, crepes, etc.
*Drinks with gluten like beer, flavored coffee, wine coolers, vodka
*Common dry breakfast cereals
*Some cheeses - blue cheese, most cottage cheese, Roquefort, Gorgonzola cheese
*Food additives - thickeners, coloring, flavoring etc.
*Energy bars
*Protein bars
*Meal replacement bars
*Breaded meats
*Processed meats
*Sauces, gravy, salad dressing
*Seasonings, desserts and snacks
*Soups - canned and mixes
*Packaged vegetarian and soy meals and products
*Malt syrup, barley extract, barley malt, malt

Flours

*All wheat flours
*Rice, corn, tapioca and potato starch
*Quinoa flour, millet flour, chestnut flour

Bad Oils

*Hydrogenated oils
*Polyunsaturated oils
*All fried foods

Sweets

*Dried fruit
*Candies, ice-cream, cakes, pastries, etc.
*Honey, maple syrup, corn syrup, etc.
*Soda
*Sugary condiments - ketchup, barbecue sauce

Food Wrap

*BPA

FIRST STEP - Get yours system off wheat, then test the waters with limited amounts of quinoa, chia, beans and millet.

Red wine on occasion is okay, but steer clear of beer!

Shortcoming One - The Wheat Belly Diet eating strategy sure is a shocker to your system. It eliminates a whole whack of foods you're accustom to eating. Which means you're going to have to dedicate more time to shop for healthy wheat-free foods, and give yourself plenty of time to adjust.

And remember, just because a product boasts gluten-free, doesn't mean it's healthy for you. Train yourself to start reading the labels and registering the less ingredients the better!

Shortcoming Two - Exercising may be mentioned on the side. But Davis fails to emphasis the importance of regular intense interval training to help lose weight and sustain weight loss. Likely because of his theory that people don't get fat because they don't exercise. Which of course we've easily already scientifically shredded.

According to *Centers for Disease Control and Prevention*, adults 17-69, need at least...

41

2.5 hours of moderate level aerobic activity each week, and muscle strength-training exercise at least two days a week, working hips, back, legs, chest, shoulders, abs, and arms.

OR

75 minutes intense cardiovascular activity each week, and at least two days a week muscle strength-training exercise.

Shortcoming Three - For the average person this is a freakin strict eating strategy. Not to say you can't make it successful. You just first need to figure out your tolerance and preferences, and only commit to the Wheat Belly Diet if you can handle it!

My Thoughts...

I've studied and experimented with oodles of different diets. And to date, I'd say the Wheat Belly Diet is the most strict when it comes to what you can and can't eat. This makes sense because by taking "wheat" out of the typical North American diet, you're not left with much.

What's important is making sure you're true to you. There are a huge number of pluses for some people with this eating strategy. But it won't work for everyone. Don't let that gynormous list of food restrictions scare you off just yet. Let's look at sample meals that might just shed some more positive light on the Wheat Belly Diet concept.

Chapter Seven - Sample Wheat-Free Meals

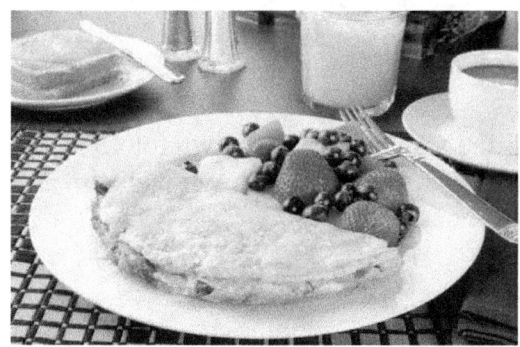

Fact - If you want to lose weight you've gotta expend more energy than you're eating. There's approximately 3500 calories in a pound. Which means you've gotta burn an extra 3500 calories to lose one pound. Experts recommend both exercising and eating less calories.

You can get some help figuring out your BMI, or how many calories your body burns at rest, from your doctor, fitness expert, or dietician. Or you can just plug your weight, height, sex, and activity level into one of the BMI calculators online yourself.

Your BMI isn't perfect, but it's a start.

Other factors affecting your BMI or Body Mass Index are:

*Genetics
*Lifestyle

*Medical condition
*Body composition

When you know how many calories your body needs, you can make an eating strategy to lose weight successfully.

For this sample eating plan, we're going to use the good old standard 2000 calorie per day diet, for a 5'6" women that's moderately active.

Note: I break the standard meals down into 3 smaller meals and 2 snacks. This helps keep energy levels up, and ensures blood sugars stay constant.

Breakfast Day 1

-2 poached eggs
-1 slice naked gluten-free wheat-free bread
-1 cup mixed berries
-Tea

Snack 1

-Grilled chicken breast wrapped in Romaine lettuce leaf
-Water

Lunch Day 1

Veggie Stir Fry - 1 cup broccoli, 1/2 cup cauliflower, 1/4 cup avocado, 1 cup spinach, 1/4 cup water chestnuts, 1/4 chicken broth, 1/4 cup sliced almonds, 1/4 cup sunflower seeds, herbs and spices to taste (warm in fry pan)
-1 cup unsweetened almond milk
-Water

Snack 2

-6-8 wheat-free specialty crackers
-1/4 cup goat cheese
-Herbal tea

Dinner Day 1

-Baked wild salmon
-1 cup green beans
-1 stalk celery with 1 tbsp. nut butter
-Water

Calories - app. 1800 calories - 50-100 grams carbs

Breakfast Day 2

-1/2 cup non-wheat gluten-free cooked cereal
-1/2 cup almond milk
-1 cup strawberries/blackberries/blueberries
-Tea
-Water with lemon

Snack 1

-1 cup Greek yogurt
-Banana
-Water

Lunch Day 2

Spinach Salad - 1 grilled 4oz steak (sliced), 6 cherry tomatoes, 1/4 cup sliced carrots, 1/4 cup sliced cucumber, sprinkler parmesan cheese, sprinkle sesame seeds
-Herbal tea
-Water

Snack 2

-2 tomatoes slices in half, topped with 2 slices turkey bacon, sprinkled with 1/4 cup shredded mozzarella cheese and broil till warm
-Water

Dinner

-1 barbecue pork chop
-1/2 cup unsweetened applesauce
-1/2 cup wild rice
-1 cup red/yellow/green/orange peppers
-Lemon water

Calories app. 2000 - 50-100 grams carbs

My Thoughts...

Even though the "no wheat" diet is very restrictive, with a little imagination and oodles of patience, you can make eating creatively tasty, healthy, and fun! These two meal days just gives you an idea of where you can start. Work with your tolerances and preferences to set yourself up for success in eating right and losing weight!

Chapter Eight - Wheat Myths and Truths

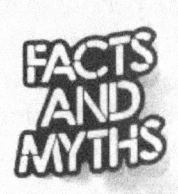

Unfortunately, what you read and hear are often distortions of the truth. These *truths* added up, can set you up for some very unhealthy eating habits, that aren't going to favor your figure.

Myth One - Wheat bread is 100% whole grain.

Truth: This is a common misconception. You can blame it on the food and drug administration if you like. Cuz it really comes down to policy. Just because wheat bread is marked on the packaging, just means there is *some* wheat in it. There might very well be 90% crap white enriched flour in the bread. Where you're almost better off having a packaged muffin!

Read the label carefully to be sure.

Myth Two - When you see *wheat-free*, that also means *gluten-free*.

Truth: Gluten is a type of protein found in *some* grains. Like wheat, barley, and rye. So you've gotta have your hawk eyes on when reading the label. Read the ingredients to make sure the product is both gluten and wheat-free, if that's what you're looking for. You know what they say when people ASSume!

Myth Three - Gluten-free is healthier for everyone.

Truth: If you're diagnosed with celiac disease, you must avoid gluten. And there are some people that have developed a sensitivity towards gluten, and may benefit from removing it from their diet. But according to *Jacksonville Florida Health and Wellness News*, make sure you get diagnosed before taking action. *There's no need to deprive yourself of a diverse range of healthy foods unnecessarily.*

Myth Four - If you chose a wheat-free diet, you're going to lose weight.

Truth: The numbers are the numbers. It doesn't matter what type of food you eat. If you're eating less calories than you're expending over a period of time, you're going to lose weight. You won't lose weight on a wheat-free diet, unless your calorie intake per day is low enough to allow weight loss.

North Florida's Department of Nutrition and Dietetics recommends not eliminating, but just reducing the serving sizes and number of servings of wheat and grain products in your diet, to aid in weight loss.

Myth Five - Gliadin is a new protein found in wheat.

Truth: Gliadin has always been around. It's a protein stored in wheat and other cereals.

Myth Six - Wheat makes you fat.

Truth: The problem of obesity in our society today is not the result of one particular type of food. That's like saying my basement flooded cuz it rained. Not true. My basement flooded because it rained, causing snow to melt faster than normal, I didn't shovel the snow out from around my house foundation. I have a crack in my foundation, and the hydro went out, so my sump pump wasn't working!

Obesity is caused by diet, genetics, health status, life style, and environment.

Myth Seven - Wheat lacks testing for health effects.

Truth: Wheat has been one of the main components of a healthy diet for thousands of years. On a global scale, it provides more than 20 percent of the total world calories, according to *Bestgrains* research.

*Wheat breeding is not a mystery. For decades breeders of wheat have been looking to improve the quality and longevity of the product safely, without sacrificing safety or nutrition. Scientific basis is valid, because it's saved zillions of lives worldwide.

What's important, is to keep an open mind, level head, and make your eating and lifestyle choices from fact, not from media hype, or one person's credentials.

My Thoughts...

I find these myths and truths quite powerful. When you've got experts questioning experts, it can get a tad confusing. My suggestion is to always search for the facts to start. And if something doesn't sit right with you, don't be afraid to question it and find the truth.

You can work to better your eating habits if you're working with truths.

Chapter Nine - Steps to Create YOUR Healthy Living Plan

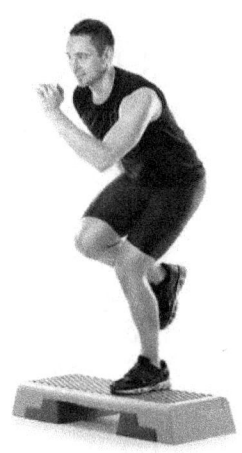

It really doesn't matter what you should and shouldn't do. What's important is creating a sustainable health plan that's effective and sustainable for YOU. Considering your preferences, tolerances, and goals.

In other words, you've gotta figure out through trial and error what works for you, and create your big picture health and wellness plan. A solid platform that will help you reach your weight loss goals and sustain them!

WebMd states having a personalized health plan increases the odds of maintaining optimal health long-term!

KISS - Here are a few steps toward healthy living...

Step One - Assess Your Current Health

This is where you need to face your reality. No judgment, blame, or regret. Just figure out where you are, mark it down, and move forward accordingly!

*Make appointments with your doctor and dentist.

*Figure out your physical measurements and calculate your BMI.

*Have a look at your daily physical activity level.

*Get a book and start writing down what you eat, where, when, why, and how much!

*Make note of your current mood and energy level in general.

*Have a look at your social circle. Is it strong and supportive with friends and family?

This is what you might call a *wake-up call*! You may not love answering all these questions, but it's your critical first step.

Recognize where you are today, so you can set healthy living goals for tomorrow!

Step Two - Prevention and Deal

By this I'm referring to dealing with current chronic health conditions you already have. Maybe you've got arthritis, high blood pressure, or pre-diabetes. Which are reason enough for you to get healthy now!

This also goes for crap habits you *know* aren't good for you. Thinks like smoking, drinking too much, partying late, and depriving yourself of sleep.

Talk with your healthcare professional or specialist to get the help you need to create a plan and take control.

Step Three - Commit to Get Physical

Here are a few pointers to slip more energy burning into your day.

*Consider your preferences and tolerances and exercise accordingly.

*Aim for 30 minutes of cardio per day, and weight training or strength training exercises 2-3 days a week, for 15 minutes each session.

Heart and Stroke Foundation of America recommends at least 180 minutes moderate to intense interval cardiovascular exercise, and at least two 15 minute sessions of diverse strength/and/or weight training exercises.

*Even if you're just taking a brisk walk around the neighborhood, it's a start!

*Every step you take matters. So mark it down in your journal, or on your phone. Check it often to remind yourself of the new actions you're taking to get healthy.

*Set yourself up for success by setting small goals. Maybe by the end of the week you want to get five bike rides in, and learn three new weight lifting exercises. Setting and resetting sensible goal is a fantabulous move!

*Something is better than zilch! Maybe you woke up late and could only fit in 15 minutes of hard biking, and 10 minutes of squats, lunges, pushups, and core work. Nothing wrong with that!

A little bit goes a long way, even if it's just to get your juices flowing and attitude programmed positive!

Step Four - Better Food Choices

I stand by my belief there is no one *perfect* diet or eating concept for anyone. Just as life always evolves, so does your body needs, lifestyle, environment, and circumstance. Add to that new health information that surfaces.

It's inevitable you're going to have to continuously assess and reassess your eating plan regularly.

Here are a few thoughts to help...

*Look at the foods you are eating and make better choices. If you're looking to cut wheat and trans fat out of your diet, instead of having a packaged vending machine muffin for breakfast and bottled juice, commit to healthier choices. Opt for 2 poached eggs, a slice of Canadian bacon, 1/2 cup of mixed berries, and a glass of water instead.

*Plan ahead by stocking the fridge and pantry with healthier foods. Prep the veggies and have them readily available, for a healthy smart snack.

*Purge the junk crap. It's much more of a jaunt to have to get dressed and head to the corner store to grab some chips. If you've got these tempting unhealthy addictive sugary foods within arm's reach, all you're going to have to do is reach.

*Learn to taste what you're eating and enjoy it. So often we're rushing through our food, not even aware of what or how much we're eating. This is learned, and can be unlearned.

Consciously slow down, chew your food, taste, and enjoy it. You'll eat less!

*Commit to eating a variety of foods. This gives you all your essential vitamins and minerals your body needs. Minus all the processed high saturated fat fast food foods!

With the Wheat Belly Diet, you're going to focus on oodles of lean protein that's grass fed, fish and seafood, organic veggies, low sugar fruits, nuts and seeds, water and tea to drink, along with almond milk or lemon water. That's a start anyway.

Step Five - Gain Control of Your Stress

Fact - Stress Kills!

Too much of it does anyway. And it would be pretty tough to find anyone that needed a little more stress to get healthy!

Find your route to deal with stress. Acknowledge it, but don't let it call your shots.

Tips to deal with stress...

*Go for a run
*Talk with a friend
*Meditate
*Go for a leisurely stroll
*Psychcentral says to step aside and breathe deeply

*Listen to music
*Go dancing
*Laugh
*Watch a movie
*Play hockey
*Do a crossword puzzle
*Avoid stress through awareness
*Sleep properly
*Learn to chill and relax
*Never run and hide from problems
*Talk to people

Step Six - Social Happiness

Your social network is very important in your big picture health plan. Psychologists at the *University of Kentucky* agree, a strong social network makes for better health.

You need family, friend, intimate, casual, virtual, and face to face relationships, to get balanced healthy.

Keep in mind that unhealthy relationships will hurt you. Get professional help if you're in a verbally or physically abusive relationship.

Step Seven - Get Proper Sleep!

Less sleep isn't better. The *National Sleep Foundation of America* suggests 7-9 hours of sleep per night for normal adults. This assumes you're getting QUALITY uninterrupted sleep.

Here are a few pointers to help you out...

*No exercising 2 hours before bed. This just gets your internal adrenalin juices flowing, which signals to your brain you're wired and ready to go!

*No stimulants like soda or coffee close to lights out, for obvious reasons.

*Teach your body your sleep routing by turning lights off, keeping the music low, and talking softer close to sleep.

*Wearing comfy clothing will help you sleep. May I suggest your birthday suit? Lol

*Turn off ALL electronics. These gadget stimulate your body and find. Making it tough to settle down to sleep.

*Take a nice warm bath. This will help you relax and fall asleep.

*Set your sleep time the same each night. Eventually your body will learn this.

*If you are having serious issues with sleep interference, like sleep apnea, insomnia, or snoring, make sure you see a sleep specialist and get it sorted out!

Final Thoughts

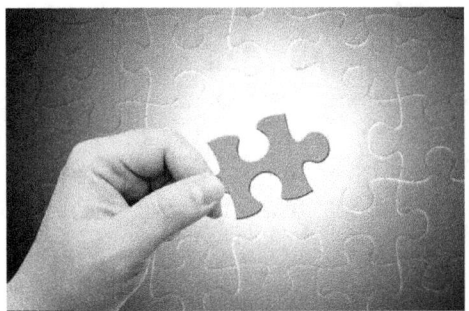

Gluten sure seems to be getting a crap rap these days. Namely due to celebrities, mass media, and self-proclaimed gluten experts.

If *Dr. Blah-Blah* wrote the book, it must be true!

If *Cameron Diaz* uses this diet to lose weight, I will too!

Are you freakin kidding me?

NOTE - The authors of these book DO NOT do their own research, or reflect on the concept personally. At least not straight-up personally. They listen to the researchers they've hired and the book gathers credentials through testimonials, NOT scientific reasoning.

FACT - Testimonials are sneaky, often fabricated, misleading, often not full-truths, and gynormously subjective.

At least with science you've got concrete facts to deal with. When someone just tells you about their belief or experience, there's a zillion influential factors you don't know about. All of which could steer them to pick the Ford Focus over Cadillac Escalade.

Case in point, is to look at all strategies with an open mind, and leave the here-say crap at the door. Start with the science of the concept, and look at the practicality, or ease of doing it. Cuz it really doesn't matter how popular the diet, or how scientifically positive it is, if you aren't going to be able to happily commit to it long term.

Can you lose weight eating wheat-free?

Absolutely!

Can you lose weight by just eating healthier and exercising regularly?

Of course you can!

If you eat a wheat-free, grain-free diet, are you going to lose weight?

Not necessarily!

Women's Health nutrition experts have some interesting points.

If you're trying to lose weight, there's not enough scientific evidence to say you'll do it eating gluten free or wheat-free. Obviously if you eat oodles of gluten filled cakes, muffins, pizza, cookies, and pasta, then you'll likely lose weight eliminating wheat.

However, there are lots of people that steer clear of this gluten protein, and are still fat.

Add to that, many gluten-free foods are loaded with blood glucose spiking sugars, have little nutrients, and are bad fat loaded, more-so than some of the wheat foods they're replacing.

To lose weight you've got to look at your eating habits, tolerances and preferences, health goals, exercise habits, general health, and lifestyle in general, in order to decide if the Wheat Belly Diet will benefit you.

Gentle Reminder - If you decide to try the Wheat Belly eating strategy, pay attention you're getting enough calcium, B vitamins, iron, zinc, vitamin D, fiber, and magnesium, cuz this diet lacks.

Focus on getting plenty of lean meat and veggies, some whole fat dairy, nuts, seeds, legumes, and fresh low glycemic index fruits. Diversity is key, and this can be pricy. Just one more factor to influence your healthy eating strategy.

Wheat Belly Diet: Grain Brain Eating is just one more concept you can use to tighten your nutrition strategy, and cinch your waistline too if you play your cards right!

Last Thoughts…

*THANK-YOU for reading my masterpiece. I hope you learned a little something, or at least got a few smiles.
*I would appreciate a millisecond or three of your time for a quick review, to help me build my masterful book empire higher.
*Whatever you do, don't forget to smile, and of course, check out my website for more of my e-Book masterpieces at:
www.flawlesscreativewriting.com

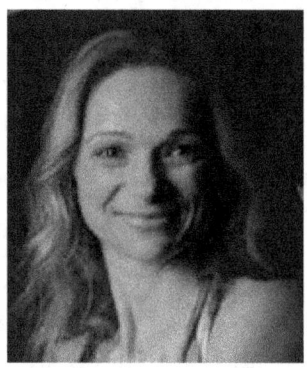

Cathy ☺

www.ingramcontent.com/pod-product-compliance
Lightning Source LLC
Chambersburg PA
CBHW060646290526
45793CB00001B/423